EAT RIGHT FOR BLOOD TYPE O

INDIVIDUAL FOOD, DRINK AND SUPPLEMENT LISTS

from

EAT RIGHT 4 YOUR TYPE

Dr. Peter J. D'Adamo
with Catherine Whitney

PENGUIN BOOKS

PENGUIN BOOKS

Published by the Penguin Group
Penguin Books Ltd, 80 Strand, London WC2R 0RL, England
Penguin Putnam Inc., 375 Hudson Street, New York, New York 10014, USA
Penguin Books Australia Ltd, 250 Camberwell Road, Camberwell, Victoria 3124, Australia
Penguin Books Canada Ltd, 10 Alcorn Avenue, Toronto, Ontario, Canada M4V 3B2
Penguin Books India (P) Ltd, 11 Community Centre, Panchsheel Park, New Delhi – 110 017, India
Penguin Books (NZ) Ltd, Cnr Rosedale and Airborne Roads, Albany, Auckland, New Zealand
Penguin Books (South Africa) (Pty) Ltd, 24 Sturdee Avenue, Rosebank 2196, South Africa

Penguin Books Ltd, Registered Offices: 80 Strand, London WC2R 0RL, England

www.penguin.com

First published in the United States of America by The Berkley Publishing Group 2002
First published in Great Britain in Penguin Books 2003
3

Every effort has been made to ensure that the information contained in this book is complete and accurate. However, neither the publisher nor the authors are engaged in rendering professional advice or services to the individual reader. The ideas, procedures, and suggestions contained in this book are not intended as a substitue for consulting with your physician. All matters regarding your health require medical supervision. Neither the authors nor the publisher shall be liable or responsible for any loss, injury or damage allegedly arising from any information or suggestion in this book. The opinions expressed in this book represent the personal views of the authors and not of the publisher.

Printed in England by Clays Ltd, St Ives plc

To Blood Type Os of the
Twenty-first Century, that you may fully realize
your remarkable heritage.

Contents

Acknowledgments

There are many people to thank, as no scientific pursuit is solitary. Along the way, I have been driven, inspired, and supported by all of the people who placed their confidence in me. In particular, I give deep thanks to my wife, Martha, for her love and friendship; my daughters, Claudia and Emily, for the joy they bring me; and my parents, James D'Adamo Sr., N.D., and Christl, for teaching me to trust in my intuition.

I am also more grateful than I can express to:

Catherine Whitney, my writer, and her partner, Paul Krafin, who have transformed complex scientific ideas into accessible principles of everyday life;

My literary agent, Janis Vallely, whose commitment and wisdom are a continuing aid and inspiration;

Amy Hertz, my editor at Riverhead/Putnam, whose

vision and care have turned the blood type science into a meaningful mainstream program;

Jane Dystel, Catherine's literary agent, whose advice has been welcome;

Heidi Merritt, whose devotion and attention to detail have brought the manuscript closer to perfection;

My staff at 2009 Summer Street for their dedication and support, and the hardworking staff at 5 Brook Street;

All of the wonderful patients who in their quest for health and happiness chose to honor me with their trust.

What Type Os Are Saying About the Diet

Lynette M., 32

"I was diagnosed as a Type II diabetic about a year ago, and controlling my blood glucose level has been a struggle, to say the least. The Type O Diet is amazing! I have tried vegetarianism in the past, and, until now, never understood why my health failed to improve, or why I failed to lose a significant amount of weight. As an overweight, diabetic African-American woman who is a single parent, full-time college student, apartment manager, and foreign-language tutor, it is imperative that I take care of myself. Now I'm excited to experience more energy and lower blood glucose levels after following the Type O diet for a mere few weeks. Also, I have eliminated indigestion, heartburn, and flatulence by simply avoiding wheat and corn products. I now eat small amounts of grains such as spelt, kamut, quinoa, buckwheat, rye, and brown rice. Generally, I follow the Type O diet to the letter. For-

tunately, it hasn't been too difficult eschewing typical African-American foods such as ham hocks and corn bread. I'm pleased to announce that I'm losing weight and feeling great!"

Steve S., 42

"Twenty-one years ago, my father died from a heart attack. Nine years ago, hoping to avoid that fate, I became a vegetarian. My diet consisted primarily of organic whole foods, and was grain based. Four years ago, I developed a potentially fatal autoimmune disease called pemphigus, in which my immune system attacks my skin. After being hospitalized, given 180 mg/day Prednisone, and released, I spent the next year and a half trying numerous traditional and naturopathic treatments. I remained a vegetarian, and I continued to take 30–40 mg per day of Prednisone. I underwent allergy tests, hair analysis, and numerous blood tests. I eventually became a raw-foods vegetarian. I got sicker. Since there is very little research done on pemphigus, I was forced to read about other autoimmune diseases. A common manifestation of chronic diseases is a phenomenon known as "blood sludge," or erythrocyte aggregation. Simply put, the red blood cells clump together, as if they are stuck together with Velcro. It was noted, by one of my doctors, that I, too, exhibited this phenomenon, but he didn't know what to do about it. Two months later, I read Eat Right 4 Your Type. *Dr. D'Adamo explains why blood sludge happens, and explains why it is food choice that causes*

it to happen. In short, a food that is healthy for one person can be detrimental to another, based on solid chemical reasons. So, it appeared that while I was doing everything right, I was not doing it right for me! Two months after deciding to choose my foods based on his plan, I started going into remission. I did this as a vegetarian. Seeing the positive results of these food choices, I reluctantly began to eat meat. That was a year ago. I am now in remission, taking no drugs or supplements, and getting healthier every day. I owe my life to Dr. D'Adamo."

Kristine S., 50

"I had reached the point where it seemed that all food was poisonous to me. I was very ill at least twice a day, and lived on Immodium to get through a day at work. I was also being treated for several other health problems. My gallbladder was removed, my high blood pressure was out of control, and I had a minimally functioning thyroid. Within a week of changing to the Type O Diet, I noticed significant improvement. All intestinal pain was eliminated. My high blood pressure and low thyroid activity were finally able to be regulated. I lost some weight, but the big change was in my general well-being and energy levels. People who had known me previously who had watched my daily struggle to find something to eat that wouldn't half kill me, and were aware of my general weakness, fatigue, and extremely low energy levels, were dumb-

founded. I became like a teenager again. I am a believer in eating right for your type and the evidence in my own life of its benefits cannot be questioned."

Martin G., 29

"I went from being barely able to do 15 push-ups to doing almost 30 in only two weeks on the Type O Diet. I feel like I am now filling my tank with the optimum fuel for my body. I was previously a fairly strict vegan for two years: lots of tofu, brown rice, veggie burgers, no dairy, but copious amounts of peanut butter and wheat. I felt sick most of the time, and I now realize that I was trying to jam a square peg into a round hole. The single greatest change in me since adopting the Type O Diet has been a marked decrease in my levels of anxiety and panic. I attribute it to the reduction of the constant fatigue I was feeling."

A Message for Type Os

Dear Type O Reader,

This special format book, Eat Right 4 Type O, *focuses on the principles and strategies of the Blood Type Diet as they apply to you. If you are new to the diet, you'll find this book to be a simple, accessible beginner's guide that will get you started on the basics. If you are already following the diet and have read the comprehensive series (*Eat Right 4 Your Type, Cook Right 4 Your Type, *and* Live Right 4 Your Type*), you'll find this book useful as a quick and portable reference guide for your diet.*

Since the introduction of the Blood Type Diet five years ago, I have received tens of thousands of testimonials from people all over the world. Many of them are from Type Os who have overcome chronic health problems, serious illnesses, or lifelong struggles with weight merely by eating and living in accordance with the genetic signals of their blood type. A growing body of research supports the conclusion that our individual differences do *matter when it comes to making strategic health and lifestyle decisions.*

I sincerely hope that you will join other Type Os who have had success with this plan. I invite you to share in experiencing the renewed sense of well-being and good health that have become reliable hallmarks of the Type O Diet.

Peter J. D'Adamo, N.D.

Important Note

The contents of this book have been abridged to provide only the most basic information concerning the Blood Type Diet. To gain the full therapeutic benefit of the diet, it is important that you read Dr. D'Adamo's complete research and prescriptive advice as it appears in his three books *Eat Right 4 Your Type, Cook Right 4 Your Type,* and *Live Right 4 Your Type*. These books include extensive details that will help you fully understand the important role your blood type plays in determining diet, exercise, health, disease, longevity, physical vitality, and emotional stability.

INTRODUCTION

The Blood Type–Diet Connection

The connection between blood type and diet is a new idea for most people, but they often find that it answers some of their most perplexing questions. We have long realized that there was a missing link in our comprehension of the process that leads either to the path of wellness or the path of disease. There had to be a reason why there were so many paradoxes in dietary studies and disease survival. Blood type analysis has given us a way to explain those paradoxes.

Blood types are as fundamental as creation itself. In the masterful logic of nature, the four blood types follow an unbroken trail from the earliest moment of human creation to the present day. They are the signatures of our ancient ancestors on the indestructible parchment of history. As Blood Type O, you carry the genetic imprint of the very first humans, the Cro-Magnon hunter-gatherers. The Type O gene enabled your ancestors to survive and thrive on a high-protein, meat-based diet. Amazingly, at the beginning of the twenty-first century, your immune and digestive systems still maintain a predisposition for foods that your Type O ancestors ate.

Your blood type is the key to your body's entire immune system, and as such is the essential defining factor in your health profile. Your blood type antigen serves as the guardian at the gate, creating antibodies to ward off dangerous interlopers. When an antibody encounters the antigen of a microbial invader, a reaction called "agglutination" (literally, gluing) occurs. The antibody attaches to the viral antigen and makes it very sticky. When cells, viruses, parasites, and bacteria are agglutinated, they stick together and clump up, which makes the job of their disposal all the easier.

But there is much more to the agglutination story. Scientists have learned that many foods agglutinate the cells of certain blood types but not others, meaning that a food that may be harmful to the cells of one blood type may be beneficial to the cells of another.

A chemical reaction occurs between your blood and the foods that you eat. This reaction is part of your genetic inheritance. We know this because of a factor called "lectins." Lectins, abundant and diverse proteins found in foods, have agglutinating properties that affect your blood. Lectins are a powerful way for organisms in nature to attach themselves to other organisms in nature. Often, the lectins used by viruses or bacteria can be blood type specific, making them a stickier pest for a person of that blood type. Furthermore, when you eat a food containing protein lectins that are incompatible with your blood type antigen, the lectins target an organ or bodily system (kidneys, liver, brain, stomach, etc.) and begin to agglutinate blood cells in that area. For example, the wheat germ lectin cross-reacts with Type O blood, targeting digestive enzymes and interfering with insulin production.

The Type O Diet is a way to restore the natural protective functions of your immune system, reset your metabolic clock, and clear your blood of dangerous agglutinating lectins. Depending on the severity of the condition, and the level of compliance with the plan, every person will realize some benefits from this diet.

THE TYPE O DIET BASICS

Type Os thrive on animal protein. The digestive tracts of all Type Os retain the memory of ancient times. The high-protein hunter-gatherer diet and the enormous physical demands placed on the systems of early Type Os probably kept most primitive humans in a mild state of ketosis—a condition in which the body's metabolism is altered. Ketosis is the result of a high-protein, high-fat diet that includes very few carbohydrates. The body metabolizes the proteins and fats into ketones, which are used in place of sugars in an attempt to keep glucose levels steady. The combination of ketosis, calorie deprivation, and constant physical activity made for a lean, mean hunting machine—the key to the survival of the human race.

Fortunately, organic and free-range meats are becoming more widely available. The success of the Type O Diet depends on your use of lean, chemical-free meats, poultry, and fish.

The Type O Diet works because you are able to follow a clear, logical, scientifically researched and certified dietary blueprint based on your cellular profile.

Your diet is organized into fourteen food groups:

Meats and Poultry

Seafood

Eggs and Dairy

Oils and Fats

Nuts and Seeds

Beans and Legumes

Grains, Breads and Pasta

Vegetables

Fruits

Juices and Fluids

Spices

Condiments

Herbs and Herbal Teas

Miscellaneous Beverages

Within each group, food is divided into three categories: HIGHLY BENEFICIAL, NEUTRAL and AVOID. Think of the categories this way:

- **HIGHLY BENEFICIAL** is a food that acts like a **MEDICINE.**
- **AVOID** is a food that acts like a **POISON.**
- **NEUTRAL** is a food that acts like a **FOOD.**

The Type O Diet includes a wide variety of foods, so don't worry about limitations. When possible, show preference for the Highly Beneficial foods over the Neutral foods, but feel free to enjoy the Neutral foods that suit you; they won't harm you and they contain nutrients that are necessary for a balanced diet.

At the top of each food category, you will see a chart that looks something like this (note that the frequency is sometimes weekly, sometimes daily):

BLOOD TYPE O		**Weekly, if your ancestry is . . .**		
	PORTION	AFRICAN	CAUCASIAN	ASIAN
All seafood	4–6 oz.	1–4 x	3–5 x	4–6 x

The portion suggestions according to ancestry are not meant as firm rules. My purpose here is to present a way to fine-tune your diet even more, using what is known about the particulars of your ancestry. Although peoples of different races and cultures may share a blood type, they don't always have the same frequency of the gene. For example, a Type A person may be AA, meaning both parents passed on the A gene, or AO, meaning only one parent passed on the A gene. Overall, people of African ancestry tend to carry the O gene more frequently than people of Caucasian and Asian ancestry. There are also geographic and cultural variations, as well as typical differences in the size and weight of various peoples. Use the refinements if you think they're helpful; ignore them if you find that they're not. In any case, try to formulate your own plan for portion sizes.

CHAPTER ONE

Meats and Poultry

BLOOD TYPE O		Weekly, if your ancestry is . . .		
	PORTION	AFRICAN	CAUCASIAN	ASIAN
Lean red meats	4–6 oz.(men)	5–7 x	4–6 x	3–5 x
Poultry	2–5 oz.(women and children)	1–2 x	2–3 x	3–4 x

Eat lean beef, lamb, turkey, chicken, or fish as often as you wish. The more stressful your job or demanding your exercise program, the higher the grade of protein you should eat. One note: If you are a Type O of African descent, emphasize lean red meats and game over fattier, more domestic choices like lamb or chicken. The gene for Type O developed in Africa, and your ancestors were the original Type Os. You'll benefit by refining your protein consumption in favor of the varieties of meat that were available to your African ancestors.

HIGHLY BENEFICIAL

Beef	Liver (calf)
Buffalo	Mutton
Heart/sweetbreads	Veal
Lamb	Venison

NEUTRAL

Chicken	Ostrich
Cornish hen	Partridge
Duck	Pheasant
Goat	Rabbit
Goose	Squab
Grouse	Squirrel
Guinea hen	Turkey
Horse	

AVOID

Bacon	Quail
Ham	Turtle
Pork	

CHAPTER TWO

Seafood

BLOOD TYPE O		Weekly, if your ancestry is . . .		
	PORTION	AFRICAN	CAUCASIAN	ASIAN
All seafood	4–6 oz.	2–4 x	3–5 x	2–5 x

Seafood, the second most concentrated animal protein, is best suited for Type Os of Asian and Caucasian Asian (Eurasian) descent, since seafood was a staple of your coastal ancestors' diet. Richly oiled cold-water fish, such as cod, herring, and mackerel, are excellent for Type Os. Fish oils are high in vitamin K, which promotes blood clotting. The inability to clot is often a problem for Type Os. Many seafoods are excellent sources of iodine, which regulates the thyroid function. Type Os typically have unstable thyroid functions, which cause metabolic problems and weight gain.

HIGHLY BENEFICIAL

Bass (all)	Shad
Cod	Sole (except gray sole)
Halibut	Sturgeon
Perch (all)	Swordfish
Pike	Tilefish
Rainbow trout	Yellowtail
Red snapper	

NEUTRAL

Anchovy	Chub
Beluga	Clam
Bluefish	Crab
Brook trout	Croaker
Bullhead	Cusk
Butterfish	Drum
Carp	Eel
Caviar	Flounder

NEUTRAL (CONTINUED)

Gray sole	**Parrot fish**
Grouper	**Pickerel**
Haddock	**Pompano**
Hake	**Porgy**
Halfmoon fish	**Rosefish**
Harvest fish	**Sailfish**
Herring (fresh)	**Salmon/Salmon roe**
Lobster	**Sardine**
Mackerel	**Scallop**
Mahimahi	**Scrod**
Monkfish	**Scup**
Mullet	**Sea trout**
Mussels	**Shark**
Opaleye fish	**Shrimp**
Orange roughy	**Smelt**
Oysters	**Snail (*Helix pomatia/* escargot)**

NEUTRAL (CONTINUED)

Sucker	Turtle
Sunfish	Weakfish
Tilapia	Whitefish
Tuna	Whiting

AVOID

Abalone	Herring (pickled)
Barracuda	Lox (smoked salmon)
Catfish	Muskellunge
Caviar	Octopus
Conch	Pollack
Frog	Squid (calamari)

CHAPTER THREE

Eggs and Dairy

BLOOD TYPE O		Weekly, if your ancestry is . . .		
	PORTION	AFRICAN	CAUCASIAN	ASIAN
Eggs	1 egg	1–4 x	3–6 x	3–4 x
Cheese	2 oz.	0–1 x	0–1 x	0–1 x
Yogurt	4–6 oz.	0–1 x	0–2 x	0–1 x
Milk	4–6 oz.	0 x	0–1 x	0–1 x

Type Os should severely restrict the use of dairy products. Your system is not designed for their proper metabolism, and there are no highly beneficial foods in this group. Eggs can be consumed in moderation. They are a good source of DHA (*Docosahexaenoic* acid), essential for mental and visual function.

If you are a Type O of African ancestry, you should eliminate dairy foods and eggs altogether. They tend to be even more difficult for you to digest; indeed, many African Americans are lactose intolerant. Soy milk and soy cheese are excellent, high-protein alternatives. Other Type Os may eat an occasional egg and have small amounts of dairy, but it is generally a poor protein source for your blood type. Be sure, however, to take a daily calcium supplement, especially if you are a woman, since dairy foods are the best natural source of absorbable calcium.

HIGHLY BENEFICIAL

None	

NEUTRAL

Butter	Feta
Egg (chicken)	Ghee (clarified butter)
Egg (duck)	Goat cheese
Farmer cheese	Mozzarella

AVOID

American cheese	Camembert
Blue cheese	Casein
Brie	Cheddar
Buttermilk	Colby

AVOID (CONTINUED)

Cottage cheese	Monterey jack
Cream cheese	Muenster
Edam	Neufchâtel
Egg (goose)	Paneer
Egg (quail)	Parmesan
Emmenthal	Provolone
Gouda	Quark cheese
Gruyère	Ricotta
Half & half	Sherbet
Ice cream	Sour cream
Jarlsberg	String cheese
Kefir	Swiss cheese
Milk (cow)	Whey
Milk (goat)	Yogurt, all varieties

CHAPTER FOUR

Oils and Fats

BLOOD TYPE O		Weekly, if your ancestry is . . .		
	PORTION	AFRICAN	CAUCASIAN	ASIAN
Oils	1 tablespoon	3–8 x	4–8 x	5–8 x

Type Os respond well to oils, which can be an important source of nutrients and an aid to elimination. You will increase their value in your system if you limit your use to the monounsaturated oils (such as olive oil) and those high in omega series fatty acids (like flaxseed oil). These oils have positive effects on the heart and arteries, and may even help reduce blood cholesterol.

HIGHLY BENEFICIAL

Linseed (flaxseed)	**Olive**

NEUTRAL

Almond	Cod liver
Black currant seed	Sesame
Borage	Walnut
Canola	

AVOID

Castor	Peanut
Coconut	Safflower
Corn	Soy
Cottonseed	Sunflower
Evening primrose	Wheat germ

CHAPTER FIVE

Nuts and Seeds

BLOOD TYPE O		Weekly, if your ancestry is . . .		
	PORTION	AFRICAN	CAUCASIAN	ASIAN
Nuts and seeds	Handful	2–5 x	2–5 x	2–4 x
Nut butters	1–2 tablespoons			

Type Os can find a good source of supplemental vegetable protein from some varieties of nuts and seeds. However, these foods should in no way take the place of high-protein meats. You certainly don't need them in your diet, and should be very selective in their use, as they are high in fat. Since nuts can sometimes cause digestive problems, be sure to chew them thoroughly, or use nut butters, which are easier to digest, especially if you have the colon problems that are more frequently experienced by Type Os.

HIGHLY BENEFICIAL

Flaxseed	Walnut (black/English)
Pumpkin seed	

NEUTRAL

Almond	Macadamia
Almond butter	Pecan
Almond cheese	Pecan butter
Almond milk	Pignola (pine nut)
Butternut	Safflower seed
Filbert (hazelnut)	Sesame butter (tahini)
Hickory	Sesame seed

AVOID

Beechnut	Peanut butter
Brazil nut	Pistachio
Cashew/butter	Poppy seed
Chestnut	Sunflower butter
Litchi	Sunflower seed
Peanut	

CHAPTER SIX

Beans and Legumes

BLOOD TYPE O		Weekly, if your ancestry is . . .		
	PORTION	AFRICAN	CAUCASIAN	ASIAN
Beans and legumes	1 cup, dry	1–3 x	1–3 x	2–4 x

Type Os of Asian ancestry utilize beans well because they are culturally accustomed to them. Even so, beans and legumes are not an important part of *any* Type O diet. That's because most beans and legumes contain lectins that deposit in the muscle tissues and make them less acidic. Try to get most of your protein from animal foods instead.

HIGHLY BENEFICIAL

Adzuki bean	**Black-eyed pea**

NEUTRAL

Black bean	Pea pod
Broad bean	Red bean
Cannellini bean	Snap bean
Fava bean	Soy bean
Garbanzo bean (chickpea)	Soy cheese*
Green bean	Soy milk*
Green pea	Soy, miso*
Jícama bean	Soy, tempeh*
Lima bean	Soy, tofu*
Mung bean (sprouts)	String bean
Northern bean	White bean

**soy products*

AVOID

Copper bean	Navy bean
Kidney bean	Pinto bean
Lentil bean	Tamarind bean

CHAPTER SEVEN

Grains, Breads and Pasta

BLOOD TYPE O		Weekly, if your ancestry is . . .		
	PORTION	AFRICAN	CAUCASIAN	ASIAN
Grains, breads, and pasta	½ cup dry grains/ pasta, 1 muffin, 2 slices bread	1–6 x	1–6 x	1–6 x

There are no grains or pastas that could be classified as highly beneficial for Type Os. Pastas made from buckwheat, Jerusalem artichoke, or rice flours are better tolerated by Type Os than the traditional semolina pasta. But these foods are not essential to your diet, and should be limited in favor of more effective animal and fish foods.

Type Os do not tolerate whole wheat products at all, and you should eliminate them completely from your diet. They contain lectins that react both with your blood and your digestive tract and interfere with the proper absorption of beneficial foods. Wheat products are a primary culprit in Type O weight gain. The glutens in wheat germ interfere with Type O metabolic processes. Inefficient or sluggish metabolism causes food to more slowly convert to energy, and so store itself as fat.

Breads and muffins can be a source of trouble for Type Os, since most of them contain some wheat flour. Two exceptions are Essene and Ezekiel bread, which are usually found in the freezer section of your local health food store. These sprouted-seed breads are assimilated by Type Os because the gluten lectins (principally found in the seed coats) are destroyed by the sprouting process. Unlike commercially-produced sprouted breads, Ezekiel and Essene breads are live foods with many beneficial enzymes intact.

HIGHLY BENEFICIAL

Essene bread (manna bread)	

NEUTRAL

Amaranth	**Ezekiel 4:9 bread (100 percent sprouted)**
Artichoke pasta (pure)	**Gluten-free bread**
Buckwheat/kasha	**Cream of Rice**

NEUTRAL (CONTINUED)

Kamut	**Rice milk**
Millet	**Rice (puffed)**
Oat bran	**Rice (white/brown/ basmati/wild)**
Oat flour	**Rye bread (100 percent)**
Oat meal	**Rye flour**
Quinoa	**Soba noodles (100 percent buckwheat)**
Puffed millet	**Soy flour bread**
Rice bran	**Spelt**
Rice bread	**Spelt flour products**
Rice cake	**Tapioca**
Rice (cream of)	**Teff**

AVOID

Barley	**Cornflakes**
Corn (white/yellow/blue)	**Cornmeal**

AVOID (CONTINUED)

Cream of Wheat	Seven grain bread/cereal
Couscous (cracked wheat)	Shredded wheat
English muffin	Sorghum
Familia	Spinach pasta
Farina	Wheat (bran)
Gluten flour	Wheat bread (sprouted commercial—not Essene/Ezekiel)
Grits	Wheat (germ)
Granola	Wheat (gluten flour products)
Grape-Nuts	Wheat (refined unbleached)
Matzo	Wheat (semolina flour products)
Popcorn	Wheat (white flour products)
Pumpernickel	Wheat (whole wheat products)

CHAPTER EIGHT

Vegetables

BLOOD TYPE 0		Daily, if your ancestry is . . .		
	PORTION	AFRICAN	CAUCASIAN	ASIAN
Cooked	1 cup, prepared	3–5 x	3–5 x	3–5 x
Raw	1 cup, prepared	3–5 x	3–5 x	3–5 x

There are a tremendous number of vegetables available to Type Os, and they form a critical component of your diet. You cannot, however, simply eat all vegetables indiscriminately. Several classes of vegetables cause big problems for Type Os. For example, certain members of the Brassica family—cauliflower, and mustard greens—can inhibit the thyroid function, which is already somewhat weaker in Type Os. Leafy green vegetables rich in vitamin K, like collards and kale, are very good for Type Os. This vitamin has one purpose only—to help blood clot. Type Os, as we have discussed, lack several clotting factors and need vitamin K to assist in the process. Alfalfa sprouts contain components that, by irritating the digestive tract, can aggravate Type O hypersensitivity problems. The molds in domestic and shiitake mushrooms, as well as fermented olives, tend to trigger allergic reactions in Type Os. All of these foods are foreign to the Type O system, which has not been designed to handle them. The nightshade vegetables, like eggplant and potatoes, cause arthritic conditions in Type Os, because their lectins deposit in the tissue surrounding your joints. Corn lectins affect the production of insulin, often leading to diabetes and obesity. All Type Os should avoid corn—especially if you have a weight problem or a family history of diabetes.

Tomatoes are a special case. Heavily laced with powerful lectins called "panhemaglutinins" (meaning they agglutinate all blood types), tomatoes are trouble for Type A and Type B digestive tracts. However, Type Os can eat tomatoes. The lectins are neutralized in your system.

HIGHLY BENEFICIAL

Artichoke	**Collard greens**
Beet greens	**Dandelion**
Broccoli	**Escarole**
Chicory	**Horseradish**

HIGHLY BENEFICIAL (CONTINUED)

Kale	Parsnip
Kelp	Pepper, red/cayenne
Kohlrabi	Potato, sweet
Lettuce, romaine	Pumpkin
Okra	Spinach
Onion, all	Swiss chard
Parsley	Turnip

NEUTRAL

Arugula	Cabbage juice
Asparagus	Carrot
Bamboo shoot	Celeriac
Beet	Celery
Bok choy	Chili pepper
Brussels sprouts	Daikon
Cabbage (Chinese/green/ red/white)	Eggplant

NEUTRAL (CONTINUED)

Endive	Rutabaga
Fennel	Sauerkraut
Fiddlehead fern	Scallion
Garlic	Shallot
Lettuce (bibb/Boston/ butter/iceberg/mesclun)	Squash (all types except pumpkin)
Mushroom (abalone/ enoki/maitake/oyster/ portobello/straw)	String bean
Olive (Greek/green/ Spanish)	Tomato/juice
Pea (green/pod/snow)	Water chestnut
Pepper (green/yellow/ jalapeno/pimiento)	Watercress
Radicchio	Yam
Radish/sprouts	Zucchini
Rappini (broccoli rabe)	

AVOID

Alfalfa sprouts	Leek
Aloe	Mustard greens
Avocado	Mushroom (shiitake/silver dollar)
Cauliflower	Olive, black
Corn	Potato (purple/red/white/yellow)
Cucumber	

CHAPTER NINE

Fruits

BLOOD TYPE O		Daily, if your ancestry is . . .		
	PORTION	AFRICAN	CAUCASIAN	ASIAN
Recommended fruits	1 cup or 1 fruit	2–4 x	3–5 x	3–5 x

Many wonderful fruits are available on the Type O Diet. Fruits are not only an important source of fiber, vitamins, and minerals, but they can also be an excellent alternative to breads and pasta for Type Os. If you eat a piece of fruit rather than a slice of bread, your system will be better served—and at the same time you'll be supporting your weight-loss goals.

Oranges and tangerines should be avoided because of their high acid content, and tendency to increase intestinal toxicity. Most other berries are okay, but stay away from blackberries, which contain a lectin that aggravates Type O digestion. Unless noted separately, all values of the whole fruits apply to their juices as well.

HIGHLY BENEFICIAL

Banana	Guava
Blueberry	Mango
Cherry (all)	Pineapple juice
Cherry juice (black)	Plum, all types
Fig (fresh/dried)	Prune

NEUTRAL

Apple	Currant (black/red)
Apple cider	Date
Apricot	Dewberry
Boysenberry	Elderberry
Breadfruit	Gooseberry
Canang melon	Grape, all types
Casaba melon	Grapefruit
Christmas melon	Kumquat
Cranberry	Lemon
Crenshaw melon	Lime

NEUTRAL (CONTINUED)

Loganberry	Prickly pear
Mulberry	Quince
Musk melon	Raisin
Nectarine	Raspberry
Papaya	Sago palm
Peach	Spanish melon
Pear	Star fruit (Carambola)
Persian melon	Strawberry
Persimmon	Watermelon
Pineapple	Youngberry
Pomegranate	

AVOID

Asian pear	Honeydew melon
Bitter melon	Kiwi
Blackberry	Orange
Cantaloupe	Plantain
Coconut/milk	Tangerine

CHAPTER TEN

Juices and Fluids

BLOOD TYPE O		Daily, if your ancestry is . . .		
	PORTION	AFRICAN	CAUCASIAN	ASIAN
Recommended juices	8 oz.	2–3 x	2–3 x	2–3 x
Water	8 oz.	4–7 x	4–7 x	4–7 x

Vegetable juices are preferable to fruit juices for Type Os because of their alkalinity. If you drink fruit juice, give preference to the low-sucrose varieties. Avoid high-sugar juices like apple juice or apple cider. Pineapple juice can be particularly helpful in avoiding water retention and bloating, both factors that contribute to weight gain. Black cherry is also a beneficial, highly alkaline juice.

Choose vegetables and fruit according to the recommendations in chapters 8 and 9 when making or buying juice.

CHAPTER ELEVEN

Spices

Your choice of spices can actually improve your digestive and immune systems. For example, kelp-based seasonings are very good for Type O because they are rich sources of iodine, key to regulating the thyroid gland. Iodized salt is another good source of iodine, but use it sparingly. The kelp bladderwrack tends to counter the hyperacidity of the Type O digestive tract, reducing the potential for ulcers. The abundant fucose in the kelp protects the intestinal lining of the Type O stomach, preventing ulcer-causing bacteria from adhering. In small amounts, sugar products such as corn syrup, honey, molasses and cane sugar will not harm you. Nor will chocolate. But these should all be strictly limited to occasional use as condiments.

HIGHLY BENEFICIAL

Carob	Kelp (bladderwrack)
Curry	Parsley
Dulse	Pepper, cayenne
Horseradish	Turmeric

NEUTRAL

Agar	Cardamom
Allspice	Chervil
Almond extract	Chili powder
Anise	Chive
Apple pectin	Chocolate
Arrowroot	Cilantro (coriander leaf)
Barley malt	Cinnamon
Basil	Clove
Bay leaf	Coriander
Bergamot	Cream of tartar
Blackstrap molasses	Cumin
Caraway	Dill

NEUTRAL (CONTINUED)

Garlic	Sage
Gelatin, plain	Savory
Honey	Sea salt
Licorice	Soy sauce
Maple syrup	Spearmint
Marjoram	Steria
Miso	Sucana
Molasses	Sugar (brown/white)
Mustard (dry)	Tamari (wheat-free)
Oregano	Tamarind
Paprika	Tapioca
Peppercorn	Tarragon
Pepper, red flakes	Thyme
Peppermint	Vanilla
Rice syrup	Vinegar (apple cider)
Rosemary	Wintergreen
Saffron	Yeast (baker's/brewer's)

AVOID

Acacia (gum Arabic)	Guarana
Algae (blue-green)	Juniper
Aspartame	Mace
Capers	Maltodextrin
Carrageenan	MSG
Corn syrup	Nutmeg
Cornstarch	Pepper (black/white ground)
Dextrose	Vinegar (except apple cider)
Fructose	
Guar gum	

CHAPTER TWELVE

Condiments

There are no highly beneficial condiments for Type Os. If you must have mustard, mayonnaise, or salad dressing on your foods, use them in moderation and stick to the low-fat, low-sugar varieties. Another option is to make your own from approved ingredients. Although Type Os can have tomatoes occasionally, avoid ketchup, as it also contains ingredients like vinegar and corn syrup. All pickled foods are indigestible for Type Os. They severely irritate the Type O stomach lining. My recommendation is that you try to wean yourself from condiments, or replace them with healthier seasonings like olive oil, lemon juice, and garlic.

HIGHLY BENEFICIAL

None	

NEUTRAL

Apple butter	Mustard (prepared, vinegar-free)
Jam (from acceptable fruits)	Salad dressing (low fat, from acceptable ingredients)
Jelly (from acceptable fruits)	

AVOID

Ketchup	Pickle, all types
Mayonnaise	Worcestershire sauce
Pickle relish	

CHAPTER THIRTEEN

Herbs and Herbal Teas

The recommendations regarding herbal teas are based on our general understanding of what makes Type Os sick. Think of herbal teas as a way to shore up your strength against your natural weaknesses. For Type Os, the primary emphasis is on soothing the digestive and immune systems. Herbs like peppermint, parsley, rose hip, and sarsaparilla all have that effect. On the other hand, herbs like alfalfa, aloe, burdock, and cornsilk stimulate the immune system and cause blood thinning, which is a problem for Type Os.

HIGHLY BENEFICIAL

Chickweed	**Fenugreek**
Dandelion	**Ginger**

HIGHLY BENEFICIAL (CONTINUED)

Hops	**Peppermint**
Linden	**Rose hip**
Mulberry	**Sarsaparilla**
Parsley	**Slippery elm**

NEUTRAL

Catnip	**Sage**
Chamomile	**Skullcap**
Dong quai	**Spearmint**
Elder	**Thyme**
Ginseng	**Valerian**
Hawthorn	**Vervain**
Horehound	**White birch**
Licorice root	**White oak bark**
Mullein	**Yarrow**
Raspberry leaf	

AVOID

Alfalfa	Red clover
Aloe	Rhubarb
Burdock	Senna
Coltsfoot	Shepherd's purse
Corn silk	St. John's wort
Echinacea	Strawberry leaf
Gentian	Yellow dock
Goldenseal	

CHAPTER FOURTEEN

Miscellaneous Beverages

There are very few acceptable beverages for Type Os. You're pretty much limited to the innocuous effects of seltzer, club soda, and herbal tea. Beer isn't recommended, as hops tend to increase stomach acid secretions and most beer is made from wheat. Modest quantities of wine are allowed, but it shouldn't be a daily ritual. Green tea is allowed as an acceptable substitute for other caffeinated products. The problem that coffee poses for Type Os is in the increased levels of stomach acid it produces. Type Os have plenty of stomach acid all their own; they really don't need help. Coffee also affects the immune system and inhibits calcium absorption. If you are a coffee drinker, perhaps you can begin to gradually cut down on the amount you consume each day. Your ultimate goal should be to eliminate drinking coffee altogether. The common withdrawal symptoms such as headache, fatigue, and irritability won't occur if you wean yourself gradually. Green tea is a good caffeinated alternative.

HIGHLY BENEFICIAL

Green tea	Seltzer water

NEUTRAL

Wine, red	

AVOID

Liquor	Tea (black regular/decaf)
Coffee (regular/decaf)	Wine, white
Soda (all types)	

CHAPTER FIFTEEN

Type O Supplement Advisory

Your Type O Plan also includes recommendations about vitamin, mineral and herbal supplements that can enhance the effects of your diet. As with food, nutritional supplements don't always work the same way for everyone. Every vitamin, mineral and herbal supplement plays a specific role in your body. The miracle remedy your Type A or Type B friend raves about may be inert or even harmful for your Type O system.

Your goal for any kind of supplementation is to enhance your Type O strengths and add an additional barrier of protection against your weaknesses. Therefore, your targeted focus should be:

- Supercharging your metabolism.
- Increasing blood-clotting activity.

- Preventing inflammation.
- Stabilizing your thyroid.

The following recommendations emphasize the supplements that help to meet these goals, and also warn against the supplements that can be counterproductive or dangerous for Type Os.

Certain common vitamins and minerals are so abundant in Type O foods that they are normally not needed in supplement form. These include vitamin C and iron—although it won't hurt you to take a 500 milligram vitamin C supplement every day. Vitamin D supplements are not needed. Many foods are vitamin D fortified, and your best source of all is the natural light of the sun. All of these recommendations are based on your adherence to the Type O Diet.

BENEFICIAL

Vitamin B

Type Os on the correct diet almost never require special vitamin B_{12} or folic acid supplementation. I have however, successfully treated depression, hyperactivity, and attention deficit disorder (ADD) in many Type Os by using high doses of folic acid and vitamin B_{12}, in conjunction with the Type O Diet and exercise program. Those vitamins are responsible for the development of DNA. If you wish to experiment with a high-potency vitamin B complex, make sure it is free of fillers and binders. Improper binding and compressing can make the pill difficult to absorb in your system. Also avoid using a formula that contains yeast or wheat germ or other avoids. Finally, eat plenty of vitamin B–rich foods.

BEST B-RICH FOODS FOR TYPE O:
meat
liver, kidney, muscle meats
eggs
fish
nuts
dark green, leafy vegetables
fruit
nutritional yeast

Vitamin K

Type Os have lower levels of several blood-clotting factors, which lead to bleeding disorders. Be sure you have plenty of vitamin K in your diet. Since it is generally not recommended as a supplement, pay attention to the foods you eat and choose those that are high in this essential Type O nutrient.

BEST K-RICH FOODS FOR TYPE O:
liver
fish oils
egg yolks
green leafy vegetables—kale and collards

Calcium

Type Os should continually supplement their diet with calcium, since the Type O Diet does not include dairy products, which are the most concentrated source of this mineral. However, with the Type O tendency to develop inflammatory joint problems and arthritis, the need for consistent calcium supplementation becomes clear. Calcium supplementation in high doses (600–1100 mg. elemental calcium) is probably desirable for all Type Os, but it is especially beneficial for Type O children during their growth periods (2–5 and 9–16), and for post-menopausal women.

Although the nondairy food sources of calcium are not as high in calcium as dairy products, Type Os should employ them as mainstays of their diets.

BEST CALCIUM-RICH FOODS FOR TYPE O:
sardines (with bones)
canned salmon (with bones)
broccoli
collard greens

Iodine

Type Os tend to have unstable thyroid metabolisms, due to a lack of iodine. This causes many side effects, including weight gain, fluid retention, and fatigue. Iodine is the only mineral that produces thyroid hormone. Although iodine supplements are not recommended, adequate amounts of iodine can be found in the Type O diet.

BEST IODINE-RICH FOODS FOR TYPE O:
seafood (especially saltwater fish)
kelp (seaweed)
iodized salt

Manganese [with caution]

It is difficult for Type Os to get manganese in your diet because it is primarily found in whole grains and legumes. For the most part this isn't a problem, and manganese supplementation is rarely recommended. However, a surprising amount of chronic joint pain (especially in the lower back and knees) in Type O patients has been helped with a short period of manganese supplementation. Never do this on your own! Manganese toxicity can result from inappropriate administration, and it should only be used under a physician's supervision.

AVOID

Vitamin A

Since your blood type is prone to slower clotting, I would not recommend that Type Os take vitamin A supplements without first checking with your doctor. These supplements can enhance blood thinning. Instead, take advantage of the rich sources of vitamin A or beta-carotene in your diet.

A-RICH FOODS ACCEPTABLE FOR TYPE O:
Cold water fish
yellow, orange, and dark leafy green vegetables

Vitamin E

Likewise, I would not recommend vitamin E supplements for Type Os because they can complicate Type O tendencies toward slower blood clotting. Instead, derive vitamin E from foods in your diet.

E-RICH FOODS ACCEPTABLE FOR TYPE O:
vegetable oils
liver
nuts
leafy green vegetables

HERBS/PHYTOCHEMICALS

Licorice (*Glycyrrhiza glabra*). The high stomach acid typical of Type Os can lead to stomach irritations. Type Os also have a susceptibility to ulcers. A licorice preparation called DGL (deglycyrrhizinated licorice) can reduce your discomfort and aid healing. DGL is widely available in health-food stores as a pleasant-tasting powder or in the form of lozenges. Unlike most ulcer medicines, DGL actually heals the stomach lining in addition to protecting it from stomach acids.

Bladderwrack (*Fucus vesiculosis*). Bladderwrack (from kelp) is an excellent nutrient for Type Os. This herb, actually a seaweed, has some interesting components, including iodine and large amounts of the sugar fucose. As you may recall, fucose is the basic building sugar of the O antigen. The fucose found in bladderwrack helps to protect the intestinal lining of Type Os—especially from the ulcer-causing bacteria, *H. pylori,* which attaches itself to the fucose lining the stomach of Type Os. The fucose in bladderwrack acts on *H. pylori* much as dust would on a piece of adhesive tape: it clogs the suction cups on the bacteria, preventing it from attaching to the stomach.

I have also found that bladderwrack is very effective as an aid to weight control for Type Os—especially those who suffer thyroid dysfunctions. The fucose in bladderwrack seems to help normalize the sluggish metabolic rate and produce weight loss.

Pancreatic enzymes. If you are a Type O who is not used to a high protein diet, I suggest you take a pancreatic enzyme along with meals until your system begins to adjust to the more concentrated proteins. Pancreatic enzyme supplements are available at most health-food stores.

CHAPTER SIXTEEN

Medical Strategies

Modern science has presented the medical community with a bewildering array of medications, and all of them are being prescribed by well-meaning physicians world-wide. But have we been careful enough in our use of an-tibiotics and vaccines? How do you know which medications are best for you, for your family, for your children? Again, blood type holds the answer.

As a naturopathic physician, I try to avoid prescribing over-the-counter medications. In most cases, there are natural alternatives that work just as well or better—and they don't have some of the problematic side effects of many pharmaceutical preparations.

The following natural remedies are safe for Type O:

ARTHRITIS

boswella

calcium

Epsom salt bath

rosemary tea soak

CONGESTION

licorice tea

mullein

nettle

vervain

CONSTIPATION

fiber

larch tree bark (ARA-6)

psyllium

slippery elm

COUGH

horehound

linden

CRAMPS, GAS

chamomile tea

fennel tea

ginger

peppermint tea

probiotic supplement with bifidus factor

DIARRHEA

blueberries

elderberries

***L. acidophilus* (yogurt culture)**

raspberry leaf

EARACHE

garlic-mullein-olive-oil eardrops

FEVER

feverfew

vervain

white willow bark

catnip

FLU

garlic

goldenseal

arabinogalactan

rose hip tea

HEADACHE

chamomile

feverfew

valerian

white willow bark

INDIGESTION, HEARTBURN

bladderwrack

bromelain

ginger

peppermint

MENSTRUAL CRAMPS

Jamaican dogwood

NAUSEA

ginger

licorice root tea

cayenne

SINUSITIS

fenugreek

thyme

SORE THROAT

fenugreek tea gargle

goldenseal-root-and-sage-tea gargle

TOOTHACHE

crushed-garlic gum massage

oil-of-cloves gum massage

CHAPTER SEVENTEEN

Frequently Asked Questions

Do I have to make all of the changes at once for my Type O Diet to work?

No. On the contrary, I suggest you start slowly, gradually eliminating the foods that are not good for you and increasing those that are highly beneficial. Many diet programs urge you to plunge in headfirst and radically change your life immediately. I think it's more realistic and ultimately more effective if you engage in a learning process. Don't just take my word for it. You have to "learn" it in your body. Before you begin your Type O Diet, you may know very little about which foods are good or bad for you. You're used to making your choices according to your taste buds, family traditions, and fad diet books. Chances are you are eating some foods that are good for you, but the Type O Diet provides you with a powerful tool for making informed choices every time. Once you know what your optimal eating plan is, you have the freedom to veer from your diet on occasion. Rigidity is the enemy of joy; I certainly am not a proponent of it. The Type O Diet is designed to make you feel great, not miserable and deprived. Obviously, there are going to be times when common sense tells you to relax the rules a bit—such as when you're eating at a relative's house.

I'm Blood Type O and my husband is Blood Type A. How do we cook and eat together? I don't want to prepare two separate meals.

My wife, Martha, and I have exactly the same situation. Martha is Type O and I am Type A. We find that we can usually share about two-thirds of a meal. The main difference is in the protein source. For example, if we make a stir-fry, Martha might separately prepare some chicken while I'll add cooked tofu. Or if we're eating a pasta dish, Martha might add a little cooked ground beef to her portion. It has become relatively easy for us because we are quite familiar with the specifics of each other's Blood Type Diet. I suggest you refer to the comprehensive books *Eat Right 4 Your Type* and *Cook Right 4 Your Type* for information and suggestions for living happily in multiple blood type families. I know that people often worry that there might be too many differences between blood types to make it work. But think about it. There are over 200 foods listed for each diet—many of them compatible across the board. Considering that the average person eats only about 25 foods, the Blood Type Diets actually offer more, not fewer, options.

Why do you list different portion recommendations according to ancestry?

The portions listings according to ancestry are merely refinements to the diet that you may find helpful. In the same way that men, women, and children have different portion standards, so, too, do people according to their body size and weight, geography, and cultural food preferences. These suggestions will help you get started until you are comfortable enough with the diet to naturally eat the appropriate portions. The portion recommendations also take into account specific problems that people of different ancestries tend to have with food. African Americans, for example, are often lactose intolerant, so the Type Bs among them may have to introduce these foods slowly to avoid negative reactions.

Must I eat all of the foods marked "highly beneficial"?

It would be impossible to eat everything on your diet! Think of your Blood Type Diet as a painter's palette from which you may choose colors in different shades and combinations. However, do try to reach the weekly serving numbers of the various food groups, if possible. Frequency is probably more important than the individual portions. If you have a small build, reduce the size of your portions, but maintain a regular frequency. This will ensure that the most valuable nutrients will continue to be delivered into the blood stream at a constant rate.

What should I do if an "avoid" food is the fourth or fifth ingredient in a recipe?

That depends on the severity of your condition, or the degree of your compliance. If you have food allergies, or colitis, you may want to practice complete avoidance. Many high-compliance patients avoid these foods altogether, although I think this might be too extreme. Unless you suffer from a specific allergic condition, it won't hurt most people to occasionally eat a food that is not on their diet.

Will I lose weight on the Blood Type Diet?

There are several ways to answer that question. First, most people who are overweight are eating an imbalanced diet—foods that upset metabolism, hamper proper digestion, and cause water retention. These are all factors that lead to overweight. The Blood Type Diet is the ultimate *balanced* diet, specifically tailored for you. If you follow your Blood Type Diet, your metabolism will adjust to its normal level and you'll burn calories more efficiently; your digestive system will process nutrients properly and reduce water retention. In time, perhaps a very short time, your weight will adjust accordingly. In my practice, I've found that most of my patients who have weight problems also have a history of chronic dieting. One would think that constant dieting would lead to weight loss, but that's not true if the structure of the diet and the foods it includes go against everything that makes sense for your specific blood type. In our culture, we tend to promote "one size fits all" weight-loss programs, and then we wonder why they don't work. The answer is obvious! Different blood types respond to food in different ways. For example, Type Os process bread and pasta differently than Type As, storing it as fat. Conversely, protein is metabolized efficiently by Type Os, but not by Type As. If you want to lose weight, your Blood Type Diet will tell you how.

In conjunction with the recommended exercise program, you should see results very quickly.

Do calories matter on the Blood Type Diet?

There is an adjustment period on this diet, and over time you'll be able to adjust food amounts according to your needs. It's important to be aware of portion sizes. No matter *what* you eat, if you eat *too much* of it you'll gain weight. This probably seems so obvious that it doesn't even bear mentioning. But overeating has become one of America's most difficult and dangerous health problems. Millions of Americans are bloated and dyspeptic because of the amounts of food they eat. When you eat excessively, the walls of your stomach stretch like an inflated balloon. Although stomach muscles are elastic and were created to contract and expand, when they are grossly enlarged the cells of the abdominal walls undergo a tremendous strain. If you are eating until you feel full, and you normally feel sluggish after a meal, try to reduce your portion sizes. Learn to listen to what your body is telling you.

I have heart problems and I've been told to totally avoid any fat and cholesterol. I'm Type O. How can I eat meat?

First, realize that it is grains, not meats, which are the cardiovascular culprits for Type O. This is especially interesting because almost everybody who has or is attempting to prevent heart disease is advised to go on a diet based largely on complex carbohydrates! For Type Os, a high intake of certain carbohydrates, usually wheat breads, increases the insulin levels. In response, your body stores more fat in the tissues, and fat levels are elevated in the blood. Also bear in mind that your blood cholesterol level is only moderately controlled by the dietary intake of foods that are high in cholesterol content. Approximately 85 to 90 percent is actually controlled by the manufacture and metabolism of cholesterol in your liver.

I'm Type O and don't want to eat much fat in my diet. What do you suggest?

A high-protein diet does not automatically mean one that is high in fat, especially if you avoid heavily marbleized meats. Although more expensive, try to find free-range meats that have been raised without the excessive use of antibiotics and other chemicals. Our ancestors consumed rather lean game or domestic animals that grazed on alfalfa and other grasses; today's fatty meats are produced by using high amounts of corn feed. If you can't afford or can't find free-range meats, choose the leanest cuts available and remove all excess fat before cooking. Type Os also have many other good protein choices that are naturally lower in fat—like chicken and seafood. The fat in the oil-rich fish is composed of omega-3 fatty acids, which seem to promote lower cholesterol and healthier hearts.

I've never heard of many of the grains you mention. Where do I find out more?

If you're looking for alternative grains, health-food stores are a bonanza. In recent years, many ancient grains, largely forgotten, have been rediscovered and are now being produced. Examples of these are amaranth, a grain from Mexico, and spelt, a variation of wheat that seems to be free of the problems found with whole wheat. Try them! They're not bad. Spelt flour makes a hearty, chewy bread that is quite flavorful, while several interesting breakfast cereals are now being made with amaranth. Another alternative is to use sprouted wheat breads, sometimes referred to as "Ezekiel" or "Essene" bread, as the gluten lectins found principally in the seed coat are destroyed by the sprouting process. These breads spoil rapidly and are usually found in the refrigerator cases of health-food stores. They are a "live" food, with many beneficial enzymes still intact. (Beware of commercially produced "sprouted wheat" breads, as they usually have a minority of sprouted wheat and a majority of whole wheat in their formulas.) Sprouted wheat breads are somewhat sweet tasting, as the sprouting process also releases sugars, and are moist and chewy. They make wonderful toast.

My children, ages five and seven, are reluctant to try new things. They're both Type O, and I have difficulty getting them to switch from milk to soy and from wheat to nonwheat foods. Any suggestions?

The best approach with children is to incorporate changes in a slow, gradual process. The most important area to focus on in the beginning is incorporating more of the beneficial Type O foods. Be patient about gradually reducing milk and wheat. Remember that food preferences are learned. Studies have shown that children, left to their own devices, select over the course of several weeks as good or better foods as those their parents would have picked for them. The watchwords therefore are . . . exposure to new foods and patience.

APPENDIX A

Type O at a Glance

TYPE O

The Hunter

strong · self-reliant · leader

STRENGTHS	WEAKNESSES	MEDICAL RISKS
Hardy digestive tract	Intolerant to new dietary and environmental conditions	Blood-clotting disorders
Strong immune system	Immune system can be overactive and attack itself	Inflammatory diseases, such as arthritis
Natural defenses against infections		Low thyroid production
System designed for efficient metabolism and preservation of nutrients		Ulcers
		Allergies

DIET PROFILE	WEIGHT LOSS KEY	SUPPLEMENTS	EXERCISE REGIMEN
HIGH PROTEIN Meat Fish Vegetables Fruit Limited grains, beans, legumes	AVOID Wheat Corn Navy beans Lentils Cabbage Dairy foods USE Kelp Seafood Red meat Liver Kale Spinach Broccoli Olive oil	Vitamin B Vitamin K Calcium Iodine Licorice Kelp	Intense physical exercise, such as aerobics, running, and martial arts

APPENDIX B

Blood Type Learning Center

Now that you're familiar with the basic principles of the Blood Type Diet, I encourage you to expand your level of learning and application. The "right for your type" series offers the most comprehensive, scientifically grounded, and clinically tested information available on the four blood types. In order to truly make the most of your individualized diet and lifestyle recommendations, it's important for you to have a working knowledge of all four blood types. Your differences do not exist in a vacuum, but are part of nature's complex system of opposition and synergism. Your understanding of the evolutionary factors that distinguish the blood types will enhance your ability to live more fully as a Type O. In addition, these books offer extensive additional information and recommendations about your blood type. The series includes:

Live Right 4 Your Type

The Individualized Prescription for Maximizing Health, Metabolism, and Vitality in Every Stage of Your Life

by Dr. Peter J. D'Adamo, with Catherine Whitney
(G. P. Putnam's Sons, 2001)
Also available on audiocassette

In *Live Right 4 Your Type*, Dr. D'Adamo shows how living according to blood type can help people achieve total physical and emotional health at every stage of life. Aided by cutting-edge genetic research and the documentation of hundreds of research studies, Dr. D'Adamo presents readers with a life-enhancing program, which includes:

- The latest discoveries about the genetics of blood type and how they affect the body's systems.
- A study of the role of subtypes, in particular secretor status.
- Groundbreaking data on the connection between blood type and stress, personality, and mental health.
- A thorough investigation of the variations in digestion, metabolism, and immunity, depending on blood type.

- Individualized blood type prescriptions that show how to make lifestyle adaptations, reduce stress, gain emotional balance, slow down aging, and avoid disease.
- Targeted advice for children, seniors, and women.
- Extensive research notes, patient outcomes, and resources.

Eat Right 4 Your Type

The Individualized Diet Solution to Staying Healthy, Living Longer & Achieving Your Ideal Weight

by Dr. Peter J. D'Adamo, with Catherine Whitney

(G. P. Putnam's Sons, 1996)

Also available on audiocassette

Eat Right 4 Your Type is Dr. D'Adamo's groundbreaking book, which first introduced the concept of the connection between blood type, diet, and health to a mass audience. With over two million copies in print and translated into fifty languages, *Eat Right 4 Your Type* remains the seminal work in the field. It includes:

- A detailed exploration of the anthropological and biological origins of the blood types.

- Comprehensive diet, exercise and meal plans for each blood type.
- Special recommendations for medical problems, weight loss, aging, infertility, and other issues.
- Case histories from Dr. D'Adamo's clinic, showing the remarkable results of the Blood Type Diet.
- An extensive bibliography, research and support section.

Cook Right 4 Your Type

The Practical Kitchen Companion to Eat Right 4 Your Type

by Dr. Peter J. D'Adamo, with Catherine Whitney

(G. P. Putnam's Sons, 1998)

Cook Right 4 Your Type is the essential guide for living with and enjoying your Blood Type Diet. With the assistance of a team of professional chefs, Dr. D'Adamo presents a book chock-full of vital information and delicious recipes for each blood type. The book features:

- Food lists and shopping guides to help you set up your kitchen.

- Family-friendly recipe charts that show how to cook for more than one blood type.
- Hundreds of tips and practical guidelines for eating right for your type.
- 30-day meal plans to help integrate the diet into daily life.
- More than 200 original recipes to please every blood type palate.

APPENDIX C

Resources and Support

DR. PETER J. D'ADAMO: PATIENT SERVICES

Dr. Peter D'Adamo and his staff continue to accept new patients on a limited basis. To find out more about scheduling an appointment, please contact:

The D'Adamo Clinic
2009 Summer Street
Stamford, CT 06905
203-348-4800

Note: Please do not submit questions regarding Dr. D'Adamo's work or seeking personal advice on health matters.

ON THE WEB: WWW.DADAMO.COM

The World Wide Web has proven to be a valuable venue for exploring and applying the tenets of the Blood Type Diet and lifestyle. Since January 1997 hundreds of thousands have visited the site to participate in the ABO chat groups, to peruse the scientific archives, to share experiences and recipes, and to learn more about the science of blood type. The Web site has an interactive message board and archives of past posts to the board.

One of the most important features on the Web page is the Blood Type Outcome Registry, which has facilitated the collection of data on the measurable effects of the Blood Type Diet on a wide range of medical conditions. Visitors are encouraged to share their results.

SELF-TESTING SERVICES

North American Pharmacal, Inc, is the official distributor of Home Blood Type Testing Kits. Each kit costs $7.95 and is a single-use disposable educational device capable of determining one individual's ABO and rhesus blood type. Results are obtained within four to five minutes. If you have several friends or family members who need to learn their blood type, you will need to order a separate home blood-typing kit for each individual.

All U.S. orders are shipped via UPS ground (shipping and handling cost is $5.25 per order irrespective of the number of kits ordered). Expedited shipping methods (UPS second day or next day) are available but cost more. Please contact the customer service department to inquire about rates for expedited shipping to your area.

If you are ordering a kit to be shipped outside of the U.S., shipping rates can vary dramatically and can be quite expensive. Please contact our customer service department prior to placing your order for an estimate of shipping charges for non-U.S. orders.

To order a single Home Blood Typing Kit please enclose $7.95 + $5.25 for shipping and handling and send to:

North American Pharmacal, Inc.
5 Brook Street
Norwalk, CT 06851
Tel: 203-866-7664
Fax: 203-838-4066
Toll free: 877-ABO-TYPE (877-226-8973)
www.4yourtype.com

North American Pharmacal, Inc., offers a range of other self-tests to monitor aspects of health such as stress hormone levels, female hormone levels, mineral balance, and antioxidant status. There is also a test to determine secretor status. For prices and ordering information please contact North American Pharmacal.

BLOOD TYPE PRODUCTS AND SUPPLEMENTS

North American Pharmacal, Inc., is the official distributor of Blood Type Specialty Products. The product line includes supplements, books, tapes, teas, meal replacement bars, cosmetics, and support material that makes eating and living right for your type easier. Included in this product line are: New Chapter® D'Adamo 4 Your Type Products™. These whole-food vitamins, herbs, and other food supplements have been specifically crafted to address the unique requirements of each blood type.

Also included are Sip Right 4 Your Type™ teas, Deflect™ lectin-blocking formulas, and a range of additional blood-type-specific and blood-type-friendly health products that have been formulated in partnership with The Republic of Tea and New Chapter.

Dr. Peter D'Adamo's official distributor in the UK can be contacted at:

Stacktheme Ltd
59 Bridge Street
Dollar
Scotland
FK14 7DQ

Tel: 01259 743255
Fax: 01259 743002
Email: info@stacktheme.com